Phlebotomy Manual

&

Practice Portfolio

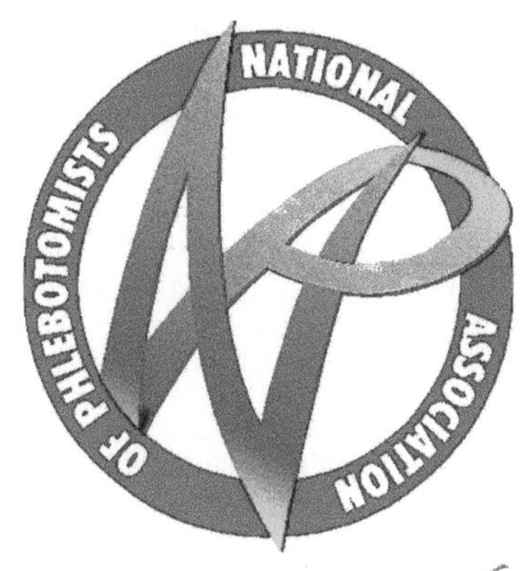

National Association of Phlebotomists

Edited by
R.F. Hoke
BSc (Hons) PG Cert HE RODP

First published in the UK 2017

Reprinted with corrections 2017

By

Firle & Rose
Portsmouth

Firle.Rose@btinternet.com

ISBN: 978-0-9933140-1-8

A catalogue record for this book is available from the British Library

Disclaimer: Whilst every effort has been taken to ensure accuracy in the contents of this text, where information differs from local policy, readers are advised to follow their employers Policies and Guidelines.

Typeset in Franklin Gothic 10.5 pt

Printed & Bound in the UK
By Lightning Source UK Ltd
Milton Keynes

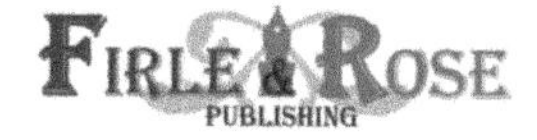

Contributing Authors

Roger Hoke (Editor)

BSc (Hons) PG Cert HE RODP — *Formerly Clinical Educator, Portsmouth Hospitals NHS Trust. Visiting lecturer, School of Health & Social Care, University of Portsmouth*

Jessie Harris

Company Secretary to National Association of Phlebotomists. Formerly, Phlebotomy Manager, Shrewsbury and Telford NHS Trust.

Jacqui Hough

Founder Member & President of the National Association of Phlebotomists. Phlebotomy Manager, Ashford & St. Peters Hospitals NHS Trust.

Cathy Williams

HNC *Medical Laboratory Science. — Founder Member and Joint President / Treasurer of the National Association of Phlebotomists. Formerly Phlebotomy Manager, Barnet & Chase Farm NHS Trust.*

About the National Association of Phlebotomists

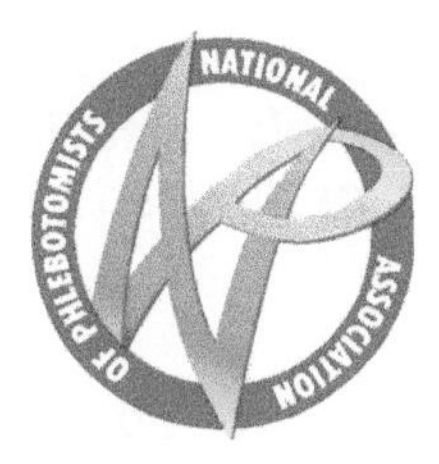

Taking phlebotomy forwards through professional recognition, the sharing of knowledge and the development of skills

The National Association of Phlebotomists was formed in 1995 with the aim of promoting national standards in phlebotomy practice to improve patient care, reduce sample errors and raise the profile of phlebotomists with recognition for this valuable skill.

National Association of Phlebotomists
Coldbath Square
London EC1R 5HL

Phlebotomy@btinternet.com
www.phlebotomy.org

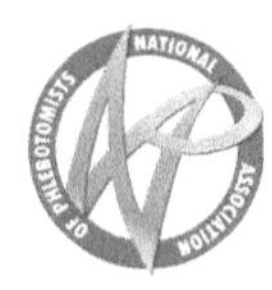

NAP Members

Code of Conduct

Members must -

- *Present as professionals, wearing uniform and a visible identification badge, as directed by local NHS Trust guidelines and policy.*
- *Introduce themselves to each patient declaring their intention.*
- *Address the patient professionally and appropriately.*
- *Explain the procedure, ensuring patient gives valid consent leaving ample opportunity for them to ask questions.*
- *Always respect the patient's need for privacy and dignity.*
- *Uphold patient confidentiality.*
- *Respect colleagues and the skill you have been trained to undertake.*

Contents

Phlebotomy Manual & Practice Portfolio

Name: ____________________

Department: ____________________

Hospital or Practice: ____________________

NAP Membership No. ____________________

Formal Training Record

Date Attended: ____/____/____

Centre: ____________________

Trainer: ____________________

Position Held: ____________________

Mentor:

Name: ____________________

Department: ____________________

Position Held: ____________________

Assessor:

Name: ____________________

Department: ____________________

Position Held ____________________

Assessment:

Date of Assessment: ____/____/____

Assessors Name: ____________________

Signature: ____________________

1. Introduction

The purpose of this manual is to provide the phlebotomist with a source of basic information to accompany the competency standards set by Skills for Health in their -

CHS132 2012 - Obtain venous blood samples

The Manual provides a toolkit to build a portfolio to record your formal training, and record how you attained and or maintain your 'Competent' status.

Completion of this manual is not a competency in itself.

Competency is confirmed by your employing authority. It will also provide a record of assessment, and serve as a portfolio of other courses attended, mandatory updates and act as a reminder of skills which need updating.

If you are new to phlebotomy, you will need some initial training. This may be a formal training course or a series of training sessions depending on your workplace.

A section at the front of the workbook provides space to record your name and workplace details, the date of your initial training, the name of your trainer, your workplace mentor and your assessor and the date of your assessment.

If you are an experienced phlebotomist wishing to build a portfolio of evidence to support your competence, you should fill in as much detail as possible using the opportunity to have your skills confirmed by your supervisor or manager. The book then becomes evidence for Continuing Professional Development (CPD).

Assessment

Ideally, your Supervisor and Assessor will be separate individuals. However, in smaller departments and in General Practice, it may be necessary for this to be the same person.

The Manual is arranged so that you are able to complete assessment in stages as your skills develop.

You may undertake practical assessment at anytime at your supervisor's discretion or following local policy.

Staff who are new to phlebotomy should be afforded a suitable period of time to learn and consolidate their skills at an appropriate level to provide quality care to the patient and to ensure their own safety prior to assessment taking place.

Self Assessment is not acceptable

How to use this book

Notes preceded by the Open Book symbol indicate what the Standard says you must know, understand or be able to do.

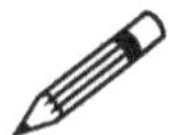

Notes preceded by the Black Pencil symbol require you to answer a question or make notes relevant to your particular practice.

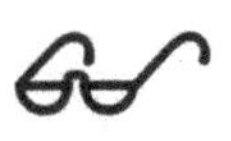

Notes preceded by the Reading Glasses symbol require you to locate and read your Department or Hospital Policy. You should sign this section when completed.

The National Association of Phlebotomists recommend that this text forms the minimum basis of all teaching and competency assessment.

2. Overview of Phlebotomy

The Standard requires you to know, understand, or are able to do -

1. The importance of positive confirmation of the patient's identity to avoid sampling errors.
2. Effective ways of gaining positive identification, following your Trust Policy.

Phlebotomy forms part of the pre-analytical phase of clinical laboratory investigations. It therefore requires that all grades of staff who collect blood samples for analysis are able to work accurately, paying particular attention to the patient's details and matching them to the blood Request Form and hospital in-patient identity Band.

Blood samples are required to –

- Confirm or eliminate a diagnosis
- Monitor effects of treatment including medication levels
- Health Screening
- Monitor disease progression
- Tissue typing

The above are important aspects of patient diagnosis, care and management. It is easy to appreciate that errors have the potential for devastating results where samples are mixed up. Every year there are 'Wrong Blood In Tube' (WBIT) reports where Patient A has a sample taken but labelled with the details of Patient B.

The Serious Hazards Of Transfusion (SHOT) Report 2015, shows a 60% rise in the number of these incidents in the last four years.

Wrong Blood In Tube (WBIT) Incidents occur where –

- **Blood is taken from the right patient but labelled with another patient's details**

Or

- **Blood is obtained from the wrong patient and labelled with the correct patient's details.**

When checking the patient's identity always use 'Open' questions which require the patient to provide the required information rather than 'Closed' questions which simply require 'yes or no' answers.

Potential Hazards of Phlebotomy

Directly - through poor technique

- Infection
- Thrombo-phlebitis
- Trauma
- Nerve damage
- Haematoma
- Arterial puncture

Indirectly - through inaccurate identification of patient or sample

- Diagnostic errors
- Treatment errors
- Death, chronic lung or kidney damage through incompatible blood transfusion.

- Phlebotomy requires a number of specific skills such as the ability to work consistently, accurately and safely.
- It requires the greatest attention to detail, good clinical and communication skills with colleagues and patients.

One of the most useful communication skills of all is listening. By actively listening and thoroughly checking details we can do much to eliminate these mistakes and greatly improve patient safety.

Objectives of Phlebotomy

1. **To correctly identify the patient – matching them to the Request Form.**
2. **Avoid introducing artefacts or pre-analytical errors.**
3. **Safe practice – avoiding needle-stick or other injuries.**
4. **Quality care – avoiding bruising and haematomas or other injury.**

Read your Trust or other Institution's - Patient Identification Policy.

Document Title:

Date: *Signature:*

From this Policy or Guideline, outline the steps in performing Positive Patient Identification.

3. Legal and Ethical Considerations

The Standard requires you to know, understand, or are able to do -

3. Have factual knowledge of current European (as applicable and national legislation including national and local policies.
4. Have a working knowledge of responsibilities and accountability.
5. Understand the importance of working within your sphere of competence.

The pleasure of being a professional with its responsibilities, require us to conduct ourselves appropriately at all times and respond to patients, their relatives or carers in a polite, courteous, and respectful manner.

At times, you may deal with patients who are confused, in a great deal of pain or who behave in a manner which can be difficult. Even so, we must conduct ourselves as professionals. The image we project to patients, visitors and colleagues is important.

To comply with the competency, you should be aware of the following pieces of European and National legislation and locate and read local policies and guidelines which affect or influence your practice.

European legislation includes

- Health and Safety (Sharp Instruments in Healthcare) Regulations 2013
- The Blood Safety and Quality Act 2005.

National legislation includes

- Health & Safety at Work Act 1974
- The Data Protection Act
- The Mental Capacity Act

National policies and guidelines may include

- NICE Guidelines
- Serious Hazards of Transfusion Reports
- Department of Health Guidelines - e.g. Identification Bands (Wristbands)
- Reports from MHRA
- Guidelines from the Health & Safety Executive (HSE)
- Public Health England.

Local Policies may include

- Information Governance
- Patient Identification Policy
- Identification Band Policy
- Infection Control Policy
- Phlebotomy Policy
- Sharps policy
- Adverse Incident Reporting Policy
- Hand-washing Policy
- Blood Culture Policy
- Blood Transfusion Policy
- Lone Worker Policy
- Clinical Waste Policy

In addition, there are other laws which are derived from common or case law (Civil Law) where judgement is based on previous court cases which set precedence.

Accountability

Accountability arises through agreements or contracts which are initiated in several ways. We are accountable to–

- The Patient
- The NHS Trust or other Employer
- Professional bodies
- The Law

The Patient

The contract or agreement with the patient begins when they give consent. We are accountable to the patient under civil law that show a *Duty of Care.*

The Hospital or Employing Authority

The employer sets up an agreement by virtue of their *Employment Contract.* Invariably this is supplemented by their local policies and guidelines.

Professional Organisations

Where the practitioner is a member of a professional organisation agreements such as a *Code of Conduct* and *Code of Practice* are established. Members are expected to follow guidelines and be of good character.

The Law

This includes *Statutory Acts* and *Criminal Law* which protects patients from being harmed or abused.

Duty of Care

Duty of Care requires that the practitioner considers the consequences of their actions and ensures that their acts or omissions do not cause a foreseeable risk of injury. Negligent acts are not deliberate but in the eyes of the law, they are foreseeable.

Vicarious Liability

The employer is the *Principle* whilst employees are their *Agents*. The hospital Trust or employer also has a *duty of care* to the patients and are responsible for all our acts and omissions.

Where wilful breaches of policy occur, the employer has a duty to initiate disciplinary action as appropriate including reporting to professional organisations.

Competence

It is important that all staff work within their level of experience and competence. Whenever in doubt, take advice from a senior colleague. Exceeding your level of competence is negligence.

As a competent professional, you are required to report any acts or omissions which may be detrimental to your patient, yourself or others.

Responsibility

Besides accountability, we have a responsibility to the public to ensure that the provision of healthcare meets acceptable standards and that staff and organisations are competent to practice. The public therefore demand that healthcare provision is regulated and where practice or standards fall below acceptable levels, health care providers can be held to account. This is regulated through a wide variety of means such as professional bodies, the Health and Safety Executive (HSE) and through Parliament.

Consent

Before undertaking any form of healthcare, the patient's permission must be sought. Legally and ethically, patients have the right to decide what happens to them. This includes, consent for physical examination, diagnostic tests and treatment. Importantly, patients must have the option to refuse.

Consent may be given verbally or non-verbally (implied consent) and is a continuous process. The patient is entitled to withdraw consent at any time. To continue after consent has been withdrawn may constitute assault and or battery.

Providing information to patients in a manner, which they can easily understand, is important to the consent process. However, consent goes beyond simply providing information. For this reason, the term *Valid consent* is more appropriate.

For consent to be valid, the patient must –

1. Be competent to make the decision.
2. Have received sufficient information to make an informed choice.
3. Not be acting under duress or influence from healthcare professionals or family.

Patients are entitled to refuse consent even for illogical reasons. This must not be taken as a sign that the patient is incompetent.

Best Interests

Where adult patients lack the ability or mental capacity to give or withhold consent for themselves, treatment may still be given if it is in the patient's 'best interests'. Best interests must take into account factors such as the wishes of the patient, religious and spiritual beliefs and their general health and well-being.

The Mental Capacity Act 2005

The purpose of this Act is to establish best practice and common law principles for those who lack mental capacity, and those who make decisions on their behalf. Generally, the Act applies to those aged 16 or over. It provides a statutory framework to empower and protect all individuals who lack the capacity to make some decisions for themselves and replaces Part 7 of the Mental Health Act 1983 and the whole of the Enduring

Powers of Attorney Act 1985.

There are five key principles which are set out in Section 1 of the Act.

1. A presumption of Capacity - all adults have the right to make their own decisions and must be assumed to have the capacity to do so until proven otherwise. It is important to remember that a person may have the capacity to make some decisions but not others.

2. Individuals must be given the opportunity and support to make their own decisions. Assumptions of mental capacity should never be made on the grounds of age or disabilities.

3. Individuals must be allowed to make unwise decisions even if the reason may seem irrational. They must not be considered to lack mental capacity simply because their view differs.

4. Where an act or decision is made for an individual you must consider their 'best interests'.

5. Any act or decision made for an individual under the terms of the Act should be the least restrictive of their basic rights and freedoms.

The Act sets out a single test for assessing capacity which protects individuals from unjustified assumptions concerning their capacity on the basis of their age, appearance or any aspect of the person's behaviour.

List any other local or national policies and guidelines that relate to, or affect your practice.

Neglect or ill-treatment of someone who lacks mental capacity is now a criminal offence and punishable by a term of up to five years' imprisonment.

Consenting Teenagers and Children

Teenagers between 16 and 18 years are presumed to have the competence to give consent for themselves. Although minors, they are entitled to the same level of confidentiality as an adult.

Dealing with Complaints

The purpose of this section is to give guidance on the handling of complaints. While complaints in general are rare, when they occur, there will always be a reason for the complaint.

Whether formal or informal, all complaints should be dealt with in a serious manner and wherever possible action should be taken to rule out future reoccurrences of a similar nature.

We are all responsible for the work we do as individuals. Complaints come in many forms, and people making complaints have a right to expect that where we fail in the service we provide, we will respond:

- Openly and honestly.
- In a timely manner.
- Apologise if necessary.
- Take appropriate action to ensure that failings do not reoccur.
- Take appropriate action.
- If a training need is identified, that training is provided .

Read your Trust or other institution's – Patient Consent Policy.

Document Title:

Date: ***Signature:***

4. Health Safety & Hygiene

The Standard requires you to know, understand, or are able to do -

6. Have a knowledge of how infection is spread and the actions which can prevent transferring infections to others.
7. Apply infection control measures when working with blood samples.
8. Understand the importance of applying Standard Precautions and the potential consequences of poor practice.

Phlebotomists should observe good personal hygiene and report for duty in a fresh, laundered uniform with arms bare below the elbow.

Uniforms not only project a professional image but also avoid the spread of infection. Uniforms should be comfortable for staff and suitable for the purpose. Trousers and tunics are often preferred by most phlebotomists.

Flat comfortable closed-toed shoes must be worn to protect staff in the event of a needle being dropped. Long hair must be tied back. Jewellery should be limited to a plain wedding band and one pair of stud earrings. Nails to be short, unvarnished with no jagged edges that could cause harm to patients. False nails must not be worn.

While working in a laboratory environment it is important not to wear the same uniform. It is advisable to wear a clean apron to prevent cross infection to both staff and patients in a ward environment. All phlebotomists must adhere to the local uniform policy of the establishment they are working in.

Eating, Drinking and Smoking

Whilst on duty the phlebotomists' hands may be a potential source of cross contamination. To reduce the risk of transferring infection from hand to mouth the following rules must be observed:

No eating or drinking on the wards or in any clinical area where blood samples are handled.

- Food and drink must not be carried on phlebotomy trays or trolleys or in the pockets of uniforms.
- No smoking in uniform or whilst on duty.
- No application of make-up.
- No licking of labels or envelopes.
- No chewing of pens, fingernails etc.
- All members of staff must endeavour to keep their hands away from their faces, hair and mouths whilst working to reduce the risk of cross contamination. If you blow your nose your hands must be washed before commencing further venepuncture.
- Hands and work surfaces are all potential sources of contamination.

Gloves

Gloves add an extra layer of protection to the skin. They do not protect from needle-stick injury but their use is mandatory in all situations when handling body fluids: blood is a body fluid. This follows the guidelines defined in Standard Precautions. Every patient is potentially high risk from blood-borne viruses and standard precautions must be followed at all times.

Importantly, wearing gloves also protects the patient from the phlebotomy staff: patients need to be protected too. A fresh pair of gloves must be worn for each patient. They must be removed when the venepuncture is complete i.e. when the wound has been dressed and the specimens bagged and waste cleared away. They must not be worn in-between bleeding patients, when answering the telephone, opening doors or handling other equipment.

Hand Hygiene

Hand washing is universally considered to be an imperative measure in infection control and prevention in all clinical settings.

Developing good hand washing practice prevents transfer of the micro-organisms that survive and multiply on human hands, and then potentially transfer to susceptible patients.

For hand decontamination in clinical areas apply 3-5 ml of soap or antiseptic preparation to wet hands and rub together five times on each rotation of the hands ensuring each surface is covered. Alternatively, 3 ml of alcohol hand rub/gel can be used on visibly clean Hands.

NAP recommends that gloves are worn for all venepuncture procedures. Always follow your Trust policy.

Gloves need to be close fitting and thin enough to ensure adequate sensitivity. They need to be comfortable to work in and it is worth trying different sizes or manufacturers to achieve a good fit.

Difficulty feeling veins can be avoided if the vein is felt for before cleaning the area and the gloves put on whilst the alcohol is allowed to dry.

When hands must be washed or gelled

- **When hands are visibly dirty.**
- **Before direct patient contact.**
- **After direct patient contact**
- **After contact with blood/body fluid.**
- **After removal of gloves.**
- **Before and after entering or leaving isolation rooms.**
- **Before handling food.**
- **Before aseptic procedure.**
- **Before any invasive procedure.**
- **Before contact with immuno - suppressed patients.**

Hand washing is the single most important measure for preventing infection. Always follow your hospital or institutions hand hygiene Policy.

Safe Use and Disposal of Sharps

The term "sharps" refers to all syringe needles, evacuated needle assemblies, winged collection needle sets, lancets and broken glass. All sharps must be disposed of in a yellow sharps box, which is specially designed for the safe disposal, storage and incineration of hazardous waste.

To reduce the chance of percutaneous injury, sharps disposal containers should be visible and recognisable. The safe disposal of a sharp requires clear vision of both the box entry and the sharp device. Care should be taken that the lid of the container is locked into place sealing the box completely around the edge. The sharps box must not be overfilled; the contents should not be tampered with under any circumstances. When the box is three-quarters full, it should be locked, dated, signed, tagged and placed at the correct collection point.

In the promotion of best practice, it is recommended that the person assembling the 'sharps' container, dates and signs the container as well as the person who seals the box. If the sharps container is to be left unattended it should be partially closed - especially overnight. Sharps boxes should not remain in use for longer than a month.

Sharps are potentially dangerous, even when clean. For this reason, clean needles must not be unsheathed until ready to pierce the vein and in clear view of the patient. Extreme care should be taken when placing the needle in the sharps box.

Safe Disposal of Non-Sharps Waste

All contaminated equipment should be disposed of in the appropriate way. All materials used during the procedure other than sharps should be disposed of as contaminated clinical waste, using a yellow clinical waste bag.

Needle Stick Injury

Needle stick injuries occur mainly as a result of poor technique. Should an injury occur, encouraged the site to bleed (but do not squeeze) by rinsing in warm, running water. The wound must be covered with a dry dressing. The incident

Read your Trust or other Institution's - Hand Hygiene Policy.

Document Title:

Date: *Signature:*

should be reported immediately to a senior member of staff, Occupational Health or Accident and Emergency Department as per Trust Policy.

Should an injury occur,

- Encourage the site to bleed (but do not squeeze).
- Wash with liquid soap in warm, running water.
- Cover with a dry dressing.
- Report immediately to a senior member of staff.
- Attend Occupational Health or the Accident and Emergency Department as per your Trust Policy.
- Complete an Adverse Incident Report.

In the event of a 'Sharps Injury' who should you contact?

Contact: ____________________

Telephone: ____________________

Health and Safety requires treating every sharp as if it is infected. It means handling and disposing of sharps correctly in accordance with local policy in order to protect yourself and others, such as laundry and portering staff and visitors including children.

Key safety procedures include:

- Wash hands before and after procedures.
- Mop up splashes and spillages.
- Cover cuts and abrasions with a waterproof dressing.
- Place sharps in a sharps container immediately after use. Containers should be out of the reach of children and as near as practicable to sites of use.
- Never overfill sharps containers. In practice this means closing and replacing them when they are three-quarters full.
- Never re-sheath a needle.

Dispose of needles and holders as a single unit. If sharps containers require assembly before use, ensure all four corners are "clicked" into place or the circular lid is pushed on all the way around. Once assembled, they must be signed and dated.

Read your Trust or other Institution's - Sharps Policy.

Document Title:

Date: *Signature:*

Note that employers must ensure adequate arrangements are in place for the safe disposal of clinical waste in the community, as well as in hospitals (Expert Advisory Group on AIDS and Advisory Group on Hepatitis, 1998).

Blood borne viruses - Immunisation

Universal or standard precautions are designed to protect against the transmission of blood-borne viruses, notably -

- **Hepatitis B (HBV)**
- **Hepatitis C (HCV)**
- **Human Immuno-Virus (HIV).**

There are, at present, no vaccines to prevent HCV and HIV infections. Immunisation against HBV is available and is the most important means by which health care workers can be protected against the virus.

The importance of Health Care Workers having the HBV vaccine cannot be over emphasised. However, it is not a substitute for good health and safety or infection control measures because it provides no protection against other blood borne viruses.

Ref: (Expert Advisory Group on AIDS and Advisory Group on Hepatitis, 1998).

Reporting and recording procedures

Staff that sustain a sharps injury and are exposed to potentially infected blood or other body fluids should report the exposure promptly. They should seek urgent advice on further management and treatment (Expert Advisory Group on AIDS and Advisory Group on Hepatitis, 1998).

Where there is a risk of acquiring a blood-borne virus, you may be offered *Post-Exposure Prophylaxis* (PEP) treatment. The Department of Health's gold standard is that you should receive this within one hour and certainly within 24 hours. It is important that you report injuries immediately.

European Directive on the Prevention from Sharp Injuries

Following a European (EU) Directive (2010/32/EU) all member states were required to bring into effect, the laws, regulations and administrative provisions to comply with the Directive by May 2013.

This required that where safety engineered devices are manufactured, they must be available to staff who ideally will be consulted in the choice of equipment ordered. Staff must be trained in the use of these devices which must -

- Be an integral part of the devices and not a separate accessory.
- Not create other safety hazards or sources of blood exposure.
- Be operated automatically or single handed wherever possible.
- Activation of the device must be identified either by an audible or tactile or visual sign.
- The device should not be easily reversible once activated.
- Activation of the safety mechanism must be convenient and allow staff to maintain Appropriate control over the procedure.
- The device must be easy to use and require little change of technique.

Each organisation should provide the necessary policies which must be followed. Where there are any concerns, these should be discussed with your manager.

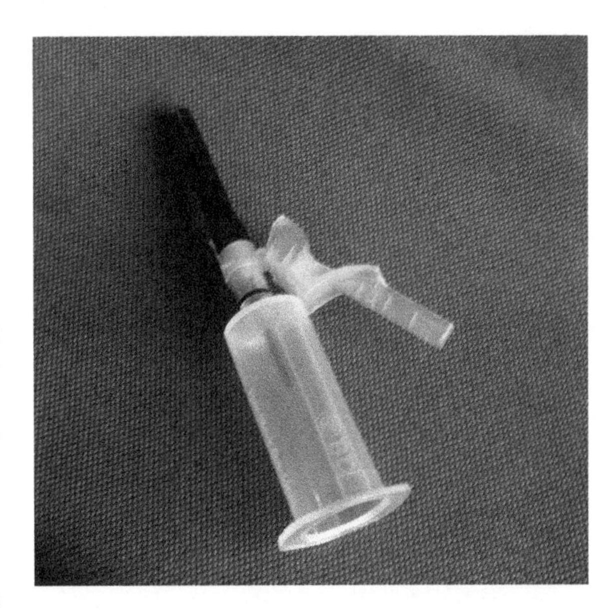

Figure 1. BD Eclipse needle showing the safety guard which lies above and in-line with the bevel of the needle.

Blood Spillage

In the event of blood spillage, the following procedure must be followed: for blood and other body fluids - do not use on chemical spills.

- Always wear appropriate personal protective clothing such as gloves and apron.
- Pour all granules over spill and leave for at least two minutes.
- Collect spill and granules mixture using scoop & scraper - discard all into the yellow disposable bag.
- Add the small tablets that are provided with spillage kit to water and carefully fill with water to the line - set aside two minutes to allow the tablets to dissolve.
- When tablets dissolve close cap and mix by inversion. Use solution with paper towels to wipe area of spill and any splashes on surrounding surfaces.
- Peel backing strip away from yellow disposable bag and stick bag to wall or table. Retain backing strip to act as tie. Place all materials, [gloves last] into the disposable bag - the bag & contents must be destroyed by incineration.

Protection by prevention is the key

All healthcare practitioners must ensure that their immunisation against Hepatitis B is up to date.

Blood Spillage Kits

Most recommended spillage kits contain -

1 X pair of disposable gloves
1 X disposable apron
1 X scoop & Scraper
1 X yellow disposal bag with tie
1 X 100 ml container of hypochlorite granules

Infection Control & Prevention

Infection may be spread by -

- Direct contact from one person to another.
- Indirectly - usually through contaminated equipment.
- Droplet - through coughs and sneezes.
- Airborne - infectious agents carried on dust.
- Ingestion - through hand to mouth contact or through contaminated food and drink.
- Vectors - such as mosquitoes.

All trays and trolleys must be cleaned daily with a hospital approved decontaminating solution. Any blood spills must be dealt with straight away. All work surfaces and phlebotomy chairs should be cleaned with a hospital approved decontamination solution at the end of each day. Spillages and splashes should be dealt with immediately.

SPECIAL REQUIREMENT ENVIRONMENTS -

Within the hospital there are areas set aside to provide special care for patients such as side rooms and isolation areas. Protocol must be adhered to whenever coming into contact with patients in these environments.

Patients in source isolation (barrier nursing)

These patients are a source of infection. They are in a single room to prevent the spread of the infection they are carrying. Gowns, gloves and sometimes masks must be worn when attending to them. Only essential equipment is taken into the room and disposable tourniquets used.

- All contaminated equipment is disposed of in the room or the lobby directly outside.
- Hands must be washed on entering and leaving. Always follow specific guidelines from your Infection Control Department.

Patients in protective isolation (reverse barrier nursing)

The patient is located in a single room that is kept as clean as possible.

All visitors are required to put on a gown or apron and gloves.

When bleeding a patient under these conditions -

- Only essential equipment is taken into the room.
- Disposable tourniquets must be used.
- Hands must be washed before entering and leaving the room.

The phlebotomist must be made aware of any special needs of the patient and abide by these during their work. Always follow specific guidelines from your infection control department.

Safety in the Environment

There are a number of basic requirements necessary to ensure that the area you are performing venepuncture in is safe:

- The patient should be seated on a chair with arms.
- The patient should not be allowed to stand to have their blood taken.
- No obstructions on the floor such as the patient's bag etc.
- Help is at hand if required.
- Patients who have a history of fainting should lie down.
- The phlebotomist is working comfortably.
- There are not too many people in the area.
- Wheelchair brakes are on.
- Patients must be sitting comfortably and safely in the chair so they do not fall should they faint.
- Immediate access to a sharps container.
- Samples are labelled and bagged correctly in the presence of the patient.
- Adequate lighting.
- Suitable flooring (no carpets).
- Adequate hand washing facilities.

Transportation of Specimens

Samples should be labelled, dated and timed in the presence of the patient. Whether in the outpatient department, wards or satellite clinics, the samples are placed in specimen bags and transported to the laboratory either by a porter, pneumatic air tube system or the phlebotomists themselves, it is essential that all samples are carried in a leak-proof container lined with absorbent material.

Samples carried in cars must be in an appropriately labelled leak-proof container. Samples posted to specialist laboratories must only be sent in approved packaging. This usually involves the sample tube being placed within a sealed screw–top plastic tube or plastic clam-shell case, wrapped in sufficient wadding to absorb the whole contents of the sample tube should a leak occur. The container is then double wrapped in sealed, leak-proof bags specially designed for the purpose.

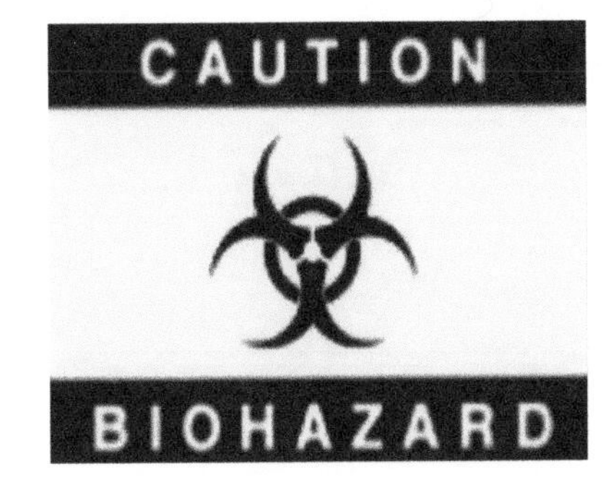

Figure 2. The standard sign used to indicate a potential bio-hazard.

Read your Trust or other Institution's - Clinical Waste Policy.

Document Title:

Date: *Signature:*

Read your Trust or other institution's - Infection Control Policy.

Document Title:

Date: *Signature:*

Read your Trust or other institution's - Health & Safety Policy.

Document Title:

Date: *Signature:*

NOTES

5. Basic Pathology

The Standard requires you to know, understand, or are able to do -

9. Select and prepare appropriate equipment including tourniquets, collection sets and sample tubes.

10. The function of different collection systems and their safety features.

Pathology is the study of disease. Pathology Departments comprise up to 8 separate areas which include Phlebotomy, Haematology, Biochemistry, Microbiology, Immunology, Mortuary, Transfusion, Histology and Cytology.

There is usually a central reception that receives all samples arriving at the department. Each sample is allocated a number; and details entered on a pathology computer then separated by centrifugation and sent to the different laboratories for testing.

Phlebotomy is associated with the pathology department and feeds almost every pathology division therefore making it a department in its own right.

Haematology

The majority of the work in this area of the laboratory is the study of red cells, white cells, and platelets. Any changes in the surface of the cells are noted as well as any changes in the total volume. Disorders, such as anaemia, haemophilia, blood clotting disorders and leukaemia are first diagnosed and then monitored in this laboratory. Staff also investigate the haemoglobin make-up found in different ethnic origins e.g. Thalassaemia.

The Coagulation section of this laboratory studies plasma and its ability to form a clot. (This may be done naturally or under the influence of various anticoagulants, - usually with an additive called sodium citrate).

Transfusion

This laboratory works with blood groups, antibodies and donor blood. This may be for transfusion or the monitoring of pregnant women. This laboratory is responsible for the selection and preparation of appropriate, compatible blood components (red blood cells, platelets and plasma) that are safe for transfusion into patients.

Blood products are also tested to check that they are free from infectious diseases such as HIV and hepatitis viruses.

Biochemistry

In this laboratory, the serum and plasma (the straw-coloured part of the blood when cellular components have been spun down) are used to measure the amount of the various chemicals and products of the metabolism present in the blood circulation.

Urine, C .S.F. (fluid taken from the spine during a lumbar puncture) and stool samples are also analysed in the biochemistry laboratory.

Microbiology

Body fluids (blood, urine, sputum, semen, C.S.F.) are usually analysed for the presence of organisms, such as bacteria, and viruses, which might cause infection. All microbiology blood tests use serum, as plasma is almost always unsuitable. The only exception to this is blood cultures where special bottles and procedures are used. Blood specimens are tested for the presence of antigens and antibodies, which may indicate evidence of past or present infection.

Immunology

This department looks at the body's defences and how the blood protects itself against infected organisms. Some of the focus is on the antibodies that the body produces to protect against recurring infections.

Cellular cytology / histology

These laboratories look at the structure of cells present in the body tissue to identify what has occurred in that part of the body. Some tissue is from "scraping" a surface to study the surface cell structure. They take tissue slices from parts of the body, mount and stain them to see what type of cells are present. They also process urine samples for cytology.

This department also deals with post–mortem examinations, biopsies, smears and the investigation into the structure of cells that are present in body tissue, to identify what has occurred in that part of the body.

Request Forms / Labelling

Request forms are generated by clinical staff and detail the tests requested for a patient. Each request form should contain the name of the consultant or requesting medical officer, the ward / department or address of the GP, also patient demographics. These must include surname, first name and date of birth. They should also include the NHS or hospital number and address where applicable.

Patients having regular anticoagulant therapy hold an prescription card that provides a record of the dosage, clotting test result and coagulation drug they are taking. The specimen should be taken to the haematology laboratory with the prescription record for the latter to be updated.

Labelling – Essential Demographics

Samples must always be labelled with details taken from the identity band in the case of an In-patient or Request form if an outpatient.

- By the person who took the sample
- In the presence of the patient
- Pre-labelled tubes must not be used.

At the time of labelling, this is the last opportunity for the patients' details to be confirmed and accurately transcribed from the request form and verified by the patient's word. This information is then labelled on the bottle which will carry the blood to the laboratory.

In order to correctly match a patient to the specimen, the phlebotomist must verify and transcribe or validate the information on the Request Form and then send the sample to the laboratory for analysis.

The laboratory will then send the report to the requesting doctor who informs, diagnoses and treats the patient. If the pre-analytical stage is compromised then the rest of the process is void, as it will only result in re- sampling the patient on another occasion.

- **ALL FORMS SHOULD BE READ VERY CAREFULLY,**
- **CHECKING DETAILS WITH THE PATIENT.**
- **DETAILS MUST ALWAYS BE TAKEN FROM THE IDENTITY BAND WHEN POSSIBLE. REMEMBER YOU HAVE INITIAL CONTACT WITH THE PATIENT AND YOUR INFORMATION MUST BE CORRECT**

There must be a minimum of four patient identifying marks, which include surname, first name and date of birth and the patient's NHS or hospital number. For auditing and specimen tracking the phlebotomist's initials must also be on each specimen as well as each request form.

In cases of time specific tests, the bottles and forms must include the date and time taken. If there is a specific instruction by the doctor e.g. fasting, the phlebotomist should indicate on the request form the date and time of the patient's last meal, and ensure the date and time of the specimen is noted on the form as well.

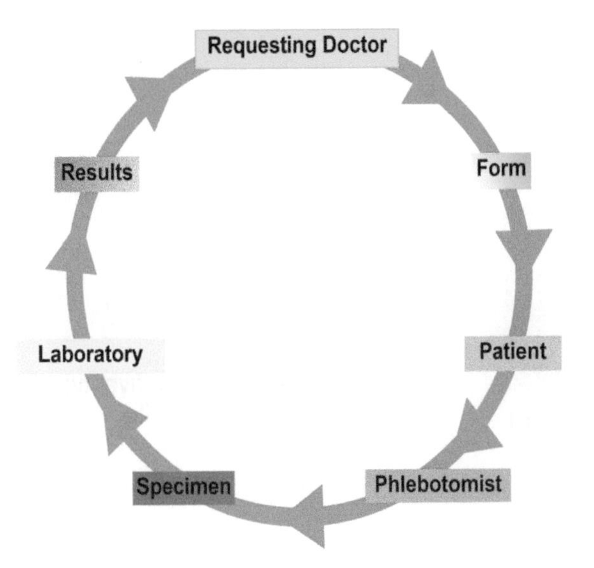

Figure 3. The cycle from the doctor requesting samples to obtaining results. This is a multi-stage process involving a number of staff with numerous opportunities for errors.

Main tests and their objectives

The following list of tests, is for background information only and not to be used to discuss tests with patients. All queries about tests and their interpretation should always be referred to the requesting doctor.

Haematology

FBC (Full Blood Count) - This test measures the number of different blood cells to detect conditions such as anaemia, infection and blood clotting disorders.

HAEMOGLOBIN. (Hb) This chemical gives the red colour to the red blood cells. It carries oxygen and contains iron. When the Hb is low the person is anaemic.

RBC - Red Blood Cell count is the number of red blood cells present. A low RBC occurs when a person has lost blood or has failed to make enough.

WBC - White Blood Cells fight bacterial infection. The count is the number of white cells present. A raised white cell count suggests infection whilst a very high count could be indicative of leukaemia which is a malignant increase in white blood cells.

Differential - There are 5 main types of white blood cells; neutrophils, lymphocytes, monocytes and eosinophils. *(See Figure 4).* It is often useful to know the proportion of each of these, and the total number of each present. The differential count will give this.

Platelets - The smallest of the blood cells, which are involved clot formation at the site of an injury.

MCV - (The size of the cells) Larger cells are present when a person lacks vitamin B12 or folate. Smaller cells are present when a person lacks iron.

ESR - Erythrocyte Sedimentation Rate. The red cells are left to settle leaving a column of plasma. The rate of settlement increases in certain illnesses, such as. arthritis and temporal arteritis.

PAUL BUNNEL (Monospot) - Paul Bunnel is a specific test for glandular fever (Infectious Mononucleosis).

Hb ELECTROPHORESIS - There are a variety of haemoglobin (Hb) molecules. A normal baby has foetal haemoglobin (Hb F) and an adult has HbA.

However, there are other Hb types. For example, those with thalassaemia, have HbA2.

If this is inherited from only one parent this is said to be thalassaemia trait. Where this is inherited from both parents it would be thalassaemia. The treatment of this disease necessitates regular blood transfusions.

SICKLE TEST - The sickle cell haemoglobin (HbS) molecule when inherited from both parents can cause red cells to become sickle shaped and cause a sickle cell crisis, which is extremely painful. When inherited from one parent, the individual is said to have sickle-cell trait. There is a quick test for HbS, but routinely Hb Electrophoresis is used.

MALARIA - The malarial parasites are identified from a blood film. This is made from the EDTA sample for FBC.

FILM - A drop of blood is spread thinly on a glass slide and stained with blue / pink stain. The shape and type of the cells are studied using a microscope.

B12/ FOLATE - When either of these components are low, it is not possible for the body to make normal red cells.

CELL MARKERS - Lymphocytes have markers on the cell surface, which can be used to identify the different types of cell. The proportion of CD3 (total lymphocytes), CD4 (helper) and CD8 (suppressor) helps in the diagnosis and monitoring of several immune conditions including HIV.

WHITE BLOOD CELLS

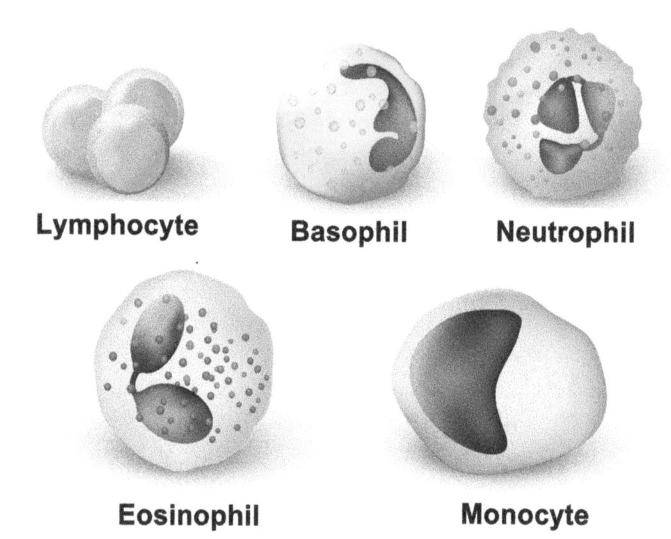

Figure 4. The five types of white blood cells.

Transfusion

GROUP AND SCREEN (RETAIN SAMPLE) - The ABO and Rh groups are carried out on the serum separated from the cells. The serum is tested for antibodies to any unusual blood groups, which could cause problems in pregnancy or in finding compatible blood. The sample is stored for a limited period in case transfusion is required.

CROSSMATCH (COMPATIBILITY) - The serum of the patient is "matched" or tested against the cells of donated blood of the same ABO and Rh group. If there is no reaction in the test it is considered that the blood is compatible with the patient, and labelled for that patient. If it is not used in 48 hours, the labels are removed and the blood placed back in stock.

ANTIBODY TITRE - An antibody titre in pregnancy could cause problems for the baby and would be monitored to see if it was getting stronger. The "titre" is the number of times the serum-containing antibody can be diluted and still show a clear reaction. For example, an antibody titre of 32 can still be detected when diluted 32 times. The higher the titre, the more risk to the baby. Antibody titre levels of 32 and above are usually serious.

GENOTYPE - If the mother has an antibody it is necessary to test the father of the child for that blood group. If he does not have the group (called antigen) there is no risk to the baby. If he is a carrier of the gene, there is a 50% risk that the baby is affected by the mother's antibody. If he has the gene the baby is at risk.

KLEIHAUER - This test is usually done on the mothers' blood to see if any baby cells are also in her circulation. They react differently to an acid solution and can be clearly seen.

DIRECT ANTIGLOBULIN TEST, DIRECT COOMBS TEST - this tests for red cells coated with antibodies on their surface. A baby affected by maternal antibody will be born with the antibody coating the red cells. Some adults make antibodies to their own cells. Coated cells only survive a few days (instead of 120).

Coagulation

APTT, KCCT, PTTK - The Activated Partial Thromboplastin time is a test for the factors at the beginning of the clotting system. It is prolonged in factor deficiencies like haemophilia (factor V111) and Christmas disease (factor 1X); this test is also used for the control of heparin anticoagulation treatment.

CLOTTING SCREEN - The clotting system consists of a series of proteins, which act together with calcium and platelets to cause a clot to form. If any of the factors are missing there is a delay in clotting which can be dangerous to the patient. A clotting screen consists of prothrombin time, thrombin time and kaolin cephalin time.

D-DIMER - This originates from the breakdown of blood clotting and is evident in cases of pulmonary embolism, deep vein thrombosis and myocardial infarction (M.I.).

FACTOR VIII assay - Other factor assays. It is possible to measure the exact level of a clotting factor for diagnosis and to check that treatment is sufficient to prevent bleeding problems.

PROTHROMBIN TIME - This is used to monitor anticoagulant treatment by Warfarin. A patient has their clotting system suppressed to fall within narrow treatment limits and is monitored regularly. The PT is reported as INR (International Normalised Ratio) which compares the patient's result with a normal control, and helps worldwide dosage.

THROMBIN TIME - This shows that there is enough fibrinogen (the basic material in a clot) and that it is functioning normally.

Biochemistry

RENAL - (Sodium, Potassium, Creatinine) - Medical staff might ask for U & E - urea and electrolytes, although creatinine has replaced urea for monitoring kidney function as it is excreted only by the glomerulus of the kidney. If necessary, urea is used to assess the patient's state of hydration. Sodium (Na) and potassium (K) are electrolytes involved in the balance of fluids inside and outside the body cells. This measurement is one of the basic standard blood tests.

LIVER - (Bilirubin, albumin, alkaline phosphatase, ALT, gamma GT) -These are liver function tests. Bilirubin is the yellow pigment from the breakdown of red cells and is raised if there is extra red cell destruction or if there is a blockage due to stones in the bile ducts which drain the liver. Albumin is a protein made by the liver and the level drops when the liver is not functioning properly. Alkaline phosphatase and ALT (alanine transaminase) are enzymes which are raised when there is liver damage. Gamma Glutamyl-transferase (gamma GT) is also used as a liver function test. This enzyme is involved in the clearance of excess alcohol or drugs and is raised in such conditions.

TROPONIN - Used to diagnose a myocardial infarction (M.I.).

PSA - Prostate specific antigen - used as a marker for prostatic carcinoma.

BONE - (alkaline phosphatase, albumin, calcium phosphate) - calcium (Ca) and phosphate (PO4) are the minerals which make up bone. The calcium result is considered together with the albumin level. Calcium levels also affect nerve function. Alkaline phosphatase (Alk phos) can also be raised when there is bone damage.

BNP - (Brain Naturetic Peptide) - a hormone in the blood which increases when heart muscle contraction becomes compromised.

CHOLESTEROL - used to estimate risk of coronary heart disease. Many laboratories agree that the patient does not need to fast unless triglycerides are being taken at same time.

GLUCOSE - Diagnosis of diabetes (fasting). Non-fasting samples for monitoring.

THYROID (TSH, Free T3, Free T4) - Thyroid stimulating hormone (TSH) is the hormone made by the pituitary gland which controls the activity of the thyroid. T3 and T4 are the hormones produced by the thyroid. (If the thyroid is not functioning properly, the levels of these hormones will alter). This would indicate whether the patient has hyper or hypo-thyroidism.

PROTEIN (Albumin, globulin) - Protein is obtained from the digestive system. If a patient is undernourished the level of protein may be low. It also drops in kidney failure when protein is lost in the urine. It may also rise in cases of severe trauma.

Laboratory Tests

Tube types often vary from laboratory to laboratory. Haematology normally require an EDTA sample for full blood counts (FBC) but may also require serum (SST) for B12, folate or citrate tubes for ESR or coagulation tests.

Biochemistry, normally requires SERUM or PLASMA sample tubes, but occasionally, may require other tubes.

Microbiology normally use plain tubes for tests other than blood cultures. Some tests are only carried out on certain days in some laboratories and may need special consideration prior to collecting the sample.

For general information on Tests and their objectives go to -

www.labtestsonline.

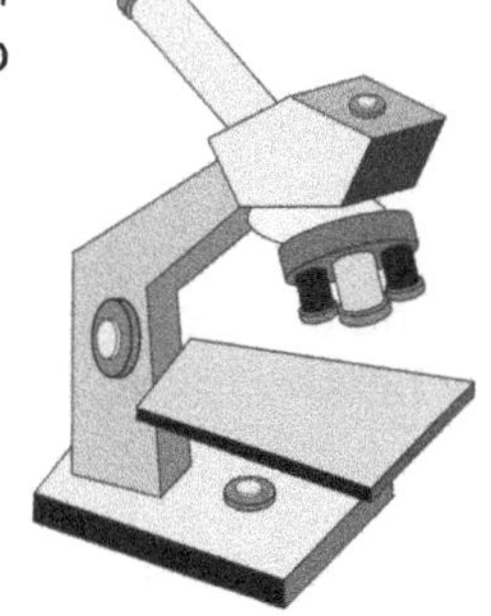

6. Anatomy & Physiology

The Standard requires you to know, understand, or are able to do -

11. Understand and know the structure of blood vessels.
12. Know the position of accessible blood vessels in relation to nerves, arteries and other anatomical structures.

The Heart

The heart is divided into two halves, left and right, separated by a muscular wall (the septum). Each half is made up of two parts; an upper chamber (the atrium) and a lower chamber (the ventricle). The upper chambers fill with blood and as their thin muscular walls contract, blood is squeezed into the lower chambers through valves which close to prevent back-flow. The *tricuspid* valve separates the upper and lower chambers of the right side of the heart and the *mitral* valve has the same function on the left side of the heart.

When the ventricles are full, the walls contract and the blood is pumped into the arteries that carry the blood from the lower chambers. The semi-lunar valves open to allow the flow of blood to the aorta, on the left and the pulmonary artery on the right. The right side of the heart sends deoxygenated blood back to the lungs for a fresh supply of oxygen. Oxygenated blood flows back to the left side of the heart through the pulmonary veins.

The movement of blood from the heart to the lungs and back again is known as pulmonary circulation. The movement of oxygenated blood from the left side of the heart to the rest of the body is known as systemic circulation.

The left ventricle, because it has to pump blood all around the body has a thicker muscular wall than the right ventricle.

Circulation of the Blood

The most important task of circulation is to carry gases and nutrients to all the tissues of the body, and to remove waste products to be filtered by organs such as the liver and kidneys.

The average adult, weighing 70 kilograms, has about 5 litres of blood in their body, which circulates through a closed system of arteries, veins and capillaries. Blood always flows in the same direction. The capillaries act as a link between the arteries and the veins.

Arteries are usually deep seated and blood passes through them under pressure. Arterial blood is oxygenated and therefore bright red in colour. It is possible to feel the beat of the heart as a pulse in the arteries.

The contraction of muscles during normal movement, squeezes the thin walled veins, aiding venous return through semi-lunar valves in the veins.

If valves are working properly, there should be no back-flow of blood.

Double Circulation

The circulatory system is divided into the venous circulation carrying de-oxygenated blood and the arterial circulation carrying oxygenated blood from the lungs.

Blood Pressure

Blood pressure rises and falls depending on how hard the heart muscle has to work. The highest blood pressure (systolic pressure) is measured when the heart muscle contracts and the blood rushes through the aorta, the main artery leaving the heart.

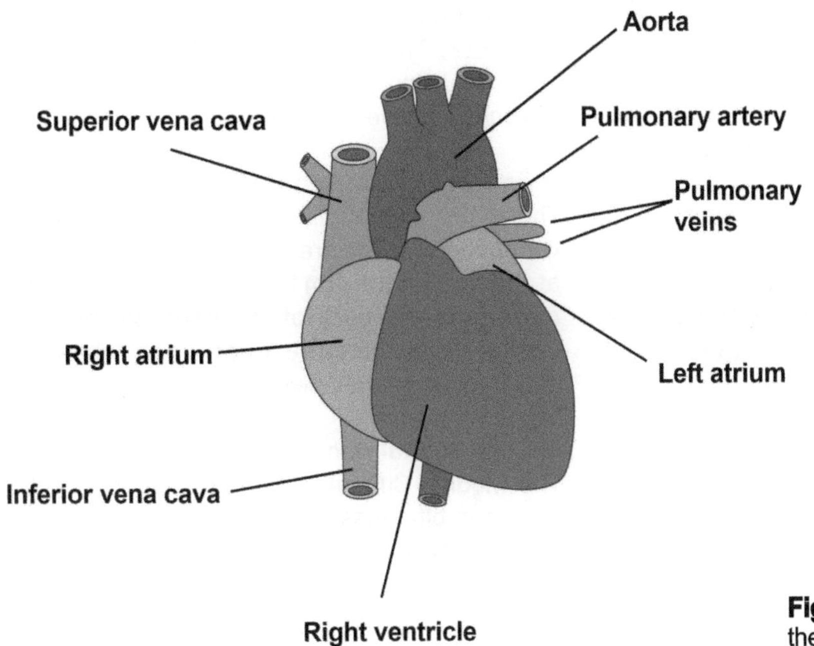

Figure 5. Diagram showing the structure of the heart.

Blood pressure is measured in millimetres of mercury [mm Hg]. The average blood pressure is 120 over 80. Systolic pressures between 100 and 140, and diastolic pressures between 70 and 90 are considered 'normal'. The instrument for recording blood pressure is called a sphygmomanometer.

Hypertension is the medical term used for high blood pressure. Patients who have hypertension should have their blood pressure checked regularly as this could result in an artery bursting and haemorrhage occurring. If blood pressure is too low, it is called hypotension.

The Blood Circulation

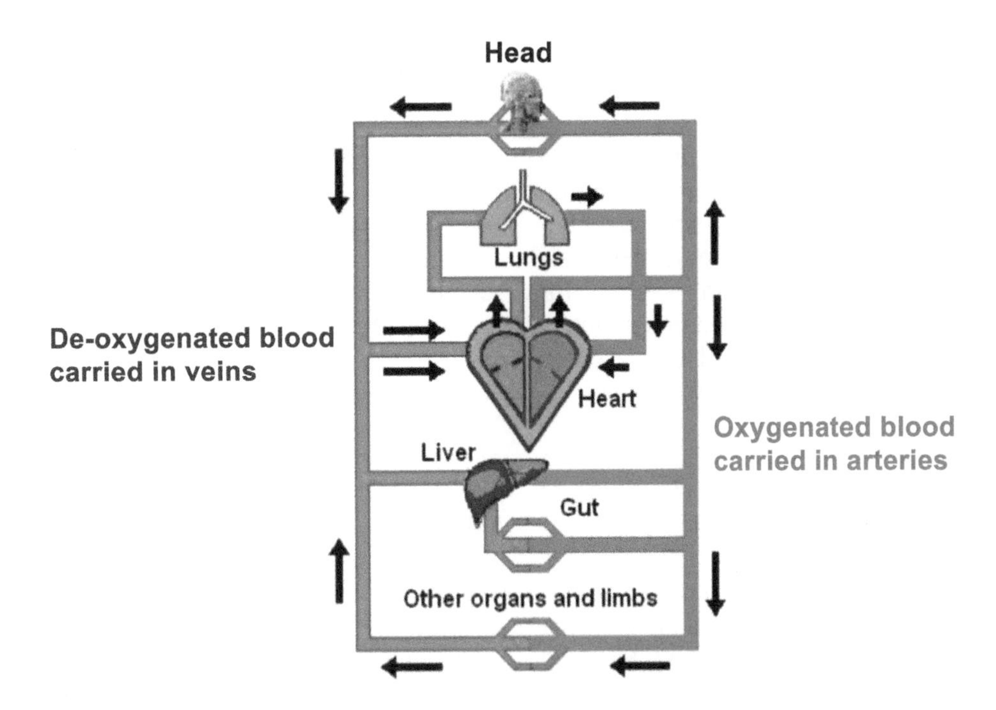

Figure 6. Diagrammatic representation of the venous and arterial circulatory systems often referred to as 'Double Circulation'.

Structure of Veins

A vein is a tube made up of three main layers;

- The ***tunica adventitia***, the outside layer, made of tough, connective tissue.
- The ***tunica media***, the middle layer made up of smooth muscle.
- The ***tunica intima***, made up of a single sheet of endothelial cells, which give a very smooth lining to the Vein.

The space through the centre of the vein where the blood flows is called the lumen. A vein has less muscle and elastic fibres in its middle layer than an artery.

Types of Veins

Veins, vary enormously among individuals and many different types will be encountered during venepuncture procedures.

Large prominent veins. These are easy to see and to feel. They are difficult to miss with the needle, but care and skill are still needed, especially with those of elderly patients whose veins are often fragile and poorly anchored.

Superficial veins. These are surface veins usually fine, dark blue in colour and easily seen. They are misleading because they are not usually substantial enough for blood collection. They bleed profusely if nicked, bruising the patient and causing discomfort.

Fine, 'thready' veins. These are not usually visible but feel like thread when palpated with the finger tips. Great care is needed when puncturing these to avoid bruising. As most hospitals have now adopted the 'closed' system for blood collection, it is recommended that a winged collection set (or 'butterfly') is used instead of the evacuated method for this type of vein.

Once a winged set is in the vein, sample tubes can be attached without the risk of the needle moving and puncturing the vein wall.

Deep veins. These are not visible and only located by palpation. They may take some time to define after the application of the tourniquet. Skill and patience are needed. However, it must be remembered that extended use of the tourniquet can result in falsely lowered potassium levels in the blood sample.

Thrombosed veins. These feel hard and knotty to the touch. There may be bruising around them. They are often found in patients who have had prolonged intravenous therapy.

Veins used in Phlebotomy

There are two main areas used for routine venepuncture. The area at the bend of the elbow at the front of the arm known as the ante-cubital fossa, and the back of the hand. In the ante-cubital fossa there are three veins which are suitable for blood collection.

Median Cubital vein.

The Median Cubital vein runs down the central part of cubital fossa area. It is well anchored by muscle and tissue and well developed in most people.

Median Cephalic vein.

This vein runs adjacent to the median cubital and runs from the midline towards the outer aspect of the arm.

Cephalic vein.

The Cephalic vein runs down the outside edge of the arm to the thumb. This vein is more mobile and may not be evident in everyone. However, it is always worth considering in difficult draws.

Basilic vein.

The Basilic vein runs from the inside edge of the arm down towards the little finger. It is often well developed. However, running in close proximity is the Brachial artery and the *internal cutaneous nerve*. It is a sensitive area and bruises easily.

The proximity of the brachial artery and the ulna nerve means that extra care must be taken when using this site in order to avoid puncturing the artery or damaging the nerve. It is best avoided for all but the most experienced staff in order to reduce the risk of permanent nerve damage.

Dorsal veins on the back of the hand

These veins should only be used by experienced phlebotomists when collection of blood from the ante-cubital fossa area is either contra-indicated or the veins are difficult to locate.

The back of the hand is a very sensitive area and skin may be quite thin. The veins are usually well developed and easily located, but extra care and skill are needed if a blood specimen is to be collected without causing bruising and haematomas. It is always recommended that a winged collection set is used.

Veins in the foot and ankle

These veins are not used routinely for the collection of blood because of the added risk of phlebitis, infection and bruising. The site however, is useful in extreme cases for example, in instances of bi-lateral mastectomy with lymph node removal.

Should it be necessary to use these veins, an appropriate size winged collection set should be used.

Each Trust will have its own guidelines on whether feet may be used by phlebotomy staff.

Factors Affecting the State of Veins

Age, clinical condition, medication and the emotional state of the patient can affect the availability of suitable veins.

Age. The veins of a young child are often difficult to find because of the presence of subcutaneous fat. In young adults and mature patients, the veins are well developed and generally easy to find. Elderly people have veins that are easily seen because the muscle tissue around them has become less stabilised and the skin may be looser. The veins are fragile and very mobile.

Clinical condition. Patients attending hospital may have to fast to undergo tests, or to have surgical procedures. They may be given drugs that affect their metabolism; they may be in pain or feeling generally ill. All these factors have an effect on the peripheral blood supply, making the location of a vein and collection of a blood specimen more difficult than usual.

Medication. Patients who are on any form of long-term medication will probably have had many blood tests to monitor drug levels. This may cause the blood vessels to become damaged and scarred. This makes the collection of blood more difficult. Patients on any form of anticoagulant therapy will be more likely to bleed excessively and to bruise.

Emotions. Attending hospital can be a very stressful experience. Patients may be apprehensive about needles or the sight of blood. They may be worried about what is wrong with them and fear bad news.

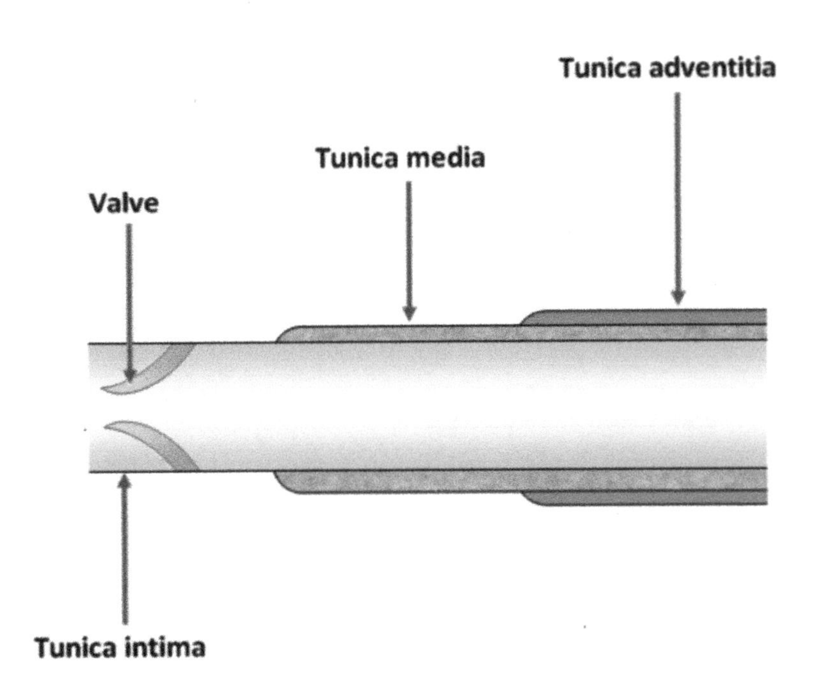

Figure 7. The structure of veins.

Fear and stress, cold and hunger can all cause the peripheral blood supply to become impaired. The veins 'disappear' and venepuncture becomes more difficult.

Nerves

These are located adjacent to the veins and often cross or pass under the vein. It is not possible to see where the nerves run and everyone will be slightly different.

For this reason, care is required when performing venepuncture. Avoid sweeping the needle around under the skin in search for a suitable vein as there is a risk of damaging or stimulating delicate nerves.

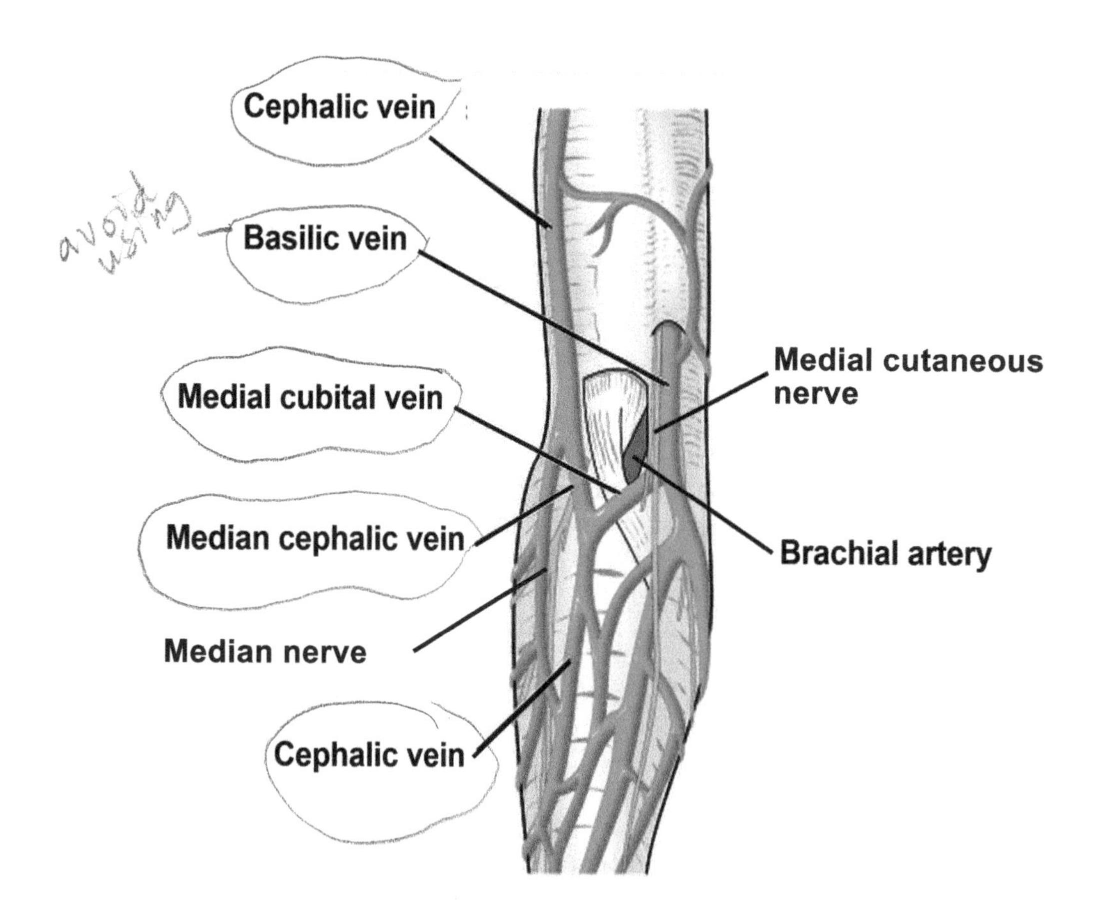

Figure 8. Diagram of Right arm showing the arrangement of veins, arteries and nerves.

<u>State the veins which are 'safe' to use</u>

1.

2.

3.

7. Phlebotomy Technique

The Standard requires you to know, understand, or are able to do -

13. How to prepare the patient.
14. The importance of correct cleansing of puncture sites.
15. The correct use of tourniquets.
16. Factors which could potentially affect the quality of the sample.
17. Recognise complications and problems when obtaining a sample and take appropriate remedial action.

The patient should be greeted with a smile and in a pleasant manner. The patient must be able to identify which phlebotomist is calling and to which cubicle to go. A way of ensuring the patient feels welcome is to meet them at the door, or at the very least to be the first person they see on entering the department. This will assist in making the patient feel welcome and possibly put them more at ease.

The phlebotomist should always face the patient whilst talking to them, ensuring eye contact. However busy the situation, the phlebotomist should show the patient that they have their full attention and concentration, for however long the procedure may take.

Identifying the Patient

The request form is checked to ensure that all relevant information has been included correctly. The patient is asked using 'open' questions to state their full name and date of birth. For example, 'What is your name please?' (surname and first name in full) and 'What is your date of birth?' (age is not sufficient).

If the name or date of birth is illegible or incorrect you should seek advice from a senior member of staff prior to obtaining a sample. You are the only point of contact with the patient from this moment so it is important that the patient is accurately identified.

Do not add tests to the form without a doctor's permission and if a doctor authorises a change make a note on the form including your initials. For patients on the ward the wristband is also required and needs to be checked as an essential method of identification.

All inpatients should be wearing a wristband. Check that the details, including the NHS or hospital number and date of birth, match those on the request forms. A positive identification must be achieved before blood is taken.

Blood must not be taken under any circumstances from in-patients who are not wearing a wristband. Contact the nursing staff for this to be remedied.

A reliable member of staff or a relative may identify a confused patient, and a record of the person identifying the patient should be made.

A patient who cannot be reliably identified should not be bled. If special conditions or preparations are required from a patient for the test, these are double-checked before venepuncture.

It is at this point that the phlebotomist should explain the procedure to the patient and obtain their consent [either verbal or implied]. Never attempt venepuncture on any patient who objects or is unsure of what is involved in the procedure.

Assessing the Arm and Selecting the most Suitable Vein

Next to correct identification of the patient, being able to select the most suitable vein is the phlebotomists' most valuable skill. It is always worth taking care to choose. Other health care professionals may need to find a 'good' vein in a hurry in an emergency, so take care to avoid injury to the patients' vessels by poor technique.

Some patients will volunteer information i.e. they will say which arm is usually the best and which vein is normally used. Some, will say why it is not possible to bleed a certain arm for whatever reason

- including mastectomy. Mostly, patients are correct about their own arms and their advice can often be useful.

- Always choose the non-dominant arm where this is possible. If necessary, check both arms to ensure that the most suitable vein is chosen.
- Gently place the patient's arm in a suitable position. If the patient is seated in a phlebotomy chair the arm should be positioned on an armrest in a straight line from the shoulder to the wrist. The arm should be very slightly flexed at the elbow.
- If the patient is in bed, have them lie on their back if possible and extend their arm. Add support under the arm with a pillow if needed.
- If the patient is seated on an ordinary chair ask them to straighten their arm, resting the back of the hand on their knee. Again, use a pillow or folded blanket for extra support.
- Ask the patient to gently close their hand (if they are able) - this usually makes veins appear more prominent.

Holding the Arm

Some patients need to be held very firmly before a venepuncture can be attempted. Patients who require assistance with holding may:

- Have a disability.
- Suffer from a disease that causes shaking e.g. Parkinson's disease.
- Be anxious and although willing, may not be able to keep still.
- Be mentally disabled and unpredictable.
- Be unable to support their arm, after a stroke for example.

Only ask someone to 'hold' if they can be relied upon to 'hold' properly. Other phlebotomists are the best people to ask as they will have been trained how and are used to doing it. The 'hold' should not be uncomfortable for the patient but should keep the arm straight for the phlebotomist performing the venepuncture and prevent the arm from bending and jerking upwards.

Never perform venepuncture on a patient who is standing up as there is always the possibility that the patient will faint and injure themselves.

Feeling for a Suitable Vein (Palpation)

Veins suitable for venepuncture should feel bouncy when palpated i.e. when the vein is pressed. Blood is squeezed out and as the vein is released, fills back up - creating the 'bouncy' feel. The vein also needs to be substantial enough to withstand the procedure.

There are 3 main veins in the bend of the elbow that are acceptable to use for venepuncture. However the *Median Cubital vein* is the vein of choice. This is usually the most prominent vein in the middle of the bend of the arm. A right-handed phlebotomist needs to feel for veins with their left hand. (The opposite is true of left-handed phlebotomists). The non-needle holding hand is used to palpate because if the vein is 'lost' during the procedure it is easier to re-locate it with the same fingers.

The tips of the middle or ring fingers are used to palpate the vein, as they tend to be more sensitive than the index finger or thumb (which also has a pulse). Initially, choose veins that are prominent and easy to palpate.

Inexperienced blood collectors lack the confidence to puncture veins that are not visible and tend to consider alternative sites but as phlebotomy skills improve, visibility is relied on less and more confidence is placed on the sense of touch.

In time, it becomes much easier to find suitable veins - experienced phlebotomists are adept at finding appropriate veins.

VEIN PALPATION - Lightly press down on the skin at the bend of the elbow repeatedly with varying degrees of pressure to detect underlying veins. Too much pressure may not allow for the tactile sensation of the vein's curvature or elasticity. Likewise, too little pressure may not bring the finger close enough to feel the vein.

Median cubital vein

This vein is usually closest to the skin's surface, which makes it easily accessible. The *Median cubital* vein tends to be well anchored in the surrounding tissue making it less likely to roll out of the way.

There is less risk of causing damage to underlying structures when this vein is used. Additionally, the surface of the skin is less sensitive over this

Median Cephalic Vein

If there is no obvious *Median Cubital vein,* the *Median cephalic* should be the next followed by the *Cephalic vein.* The latter is the occasionally prominent vein found in the ante-cubital area projecting towards to outer aspect of arm.

Cephalic Vein

This vein can be located on the outer aspect of the forearm immediately adjacent to the ante-cubital area. It can be variable in size but is often well pronounced in more muscular arms.

Basilic Vein

This vein is the last vein to be considered for venepuncture. The *Basilic vein* is situated on the inner aspect of the elbow and is often prominent on the arms of elderly patients and may be bulbous and bluish in colour. It may also be quite fragile in the elderly. If this vein is well defined and there are no other choices, it is acceptable for experienced phlebotomists to access it using a well-honed technique and a greater degree of caution - bearing in mind the extra risks of nerve damage involved.

The brachial artery and branches of the *Median Cubital antebrachial cutaneous nerve* are found in close proximity to this vein. These underlying structures may easily be damaged by careless blood collecting unless the phlebotomist proceeds with caution.

If the nerve is pierced, shooting pains will be felt down the length of the arm, from the fingers to the shoulder and the chest. If there is severe injury, nerve damage can be permanent.

Most nerve injuries resulting from venepuncture are from attempts to puncture the *Basilic vein.* Palpate the skin around the bend of the arm to distinguish between veins and other structures such as arteries and tendons.

Nerves

The main nerves of the arm are the Radial, Median, and Ulna nerves and run the full length of the arm often parallel with the veins but occasionally passing over or under the vein.

There are fewer nerves around the central veins making the *Median cubital* or *Median Cephalic* veins first choice.

Nerves cannot be seen or felt (as they are usually deep seated), but by avoiding deep probing venepunctures reduces the chance of touching a nerve considerably.

Nerve Injuries

It is rare to puncture a nerve, but if this does occur the patient may complain of severe pain, numbness or paraesthesia, or a tingling sensation. The tourniquet should be released and the needle removed immediately.

Patients often feel faint and should be laid down. They may feel sick or they may vomit. If the nerve has not been injured these symptoms will resolve; however, medical staff should be informed in case there has been permanent nerve damage. It is important to document such events and phlebotomists should follow their hospitals policy for reporting adverse incidents.

Because nerves are neither visible nor palpable, there is always a slight risk of injury during phlebotomy procedures. It is important to ensure that such injuries are not the direct result of poor technique.

Possibly the most common error leading to nerve injury is entering the vein at an excessive angle of insertion. When the needle enters the vein acutely, it is far more likely to pass through the other side of the vein than if entered at a low angle, and a greater degree of caution is required, bearing in mind the extra risks involved.

The *Basilic vein* has underlying structures that may be damaged by careless blood collecting unless the phlebotomist proceeds with caution. The brachial artery and branches of the *median cubital antebrachial cutaneous nerve* are found in close proximity to this vein.

A low angle allows a significant margin of error before emerging through the other side of the vein and potentially injuring the underlying structures. Excessive probing with a needle around the Basilic vein area can injure nerves. This vein is not as well anchored as the Median Cubital vein and it is easier to lose control of the needle. If the phlebotomist resorts to probing to access a vein the Basilic is the least forgiving.

Drawing blood from the Basilic vein brings the greatest risk to the patient because of underlying structures. Branches of the median cubital antebrachial cutaneous nerve can nestle against this vein. Once pierced, these nerves send shooting pain down the length of the limb to the fingers and up to the shoulder and chest.

If the injury is severe, nerve injury can be permanent. However, the risk is low as long as the vein is prominent. If the Median cubital vein can be accessed this is a safer area to work in. This vein should always be used if there is a choice.

The next option for consideration would be the cephalic vein. Arteries and nerves are inclined to group close to veins so care should always be taken when accessing any vein.

Arteries

Arteries pulsate when they are palpated. It is rare to puncture an artery however, if this should occur, the needle should be withdrawn and firm pressure applied on the puncture site for at least 5 minutes.

Although the *Brachial artery* is usually situated deep in the arm, great care must be taken to avoid it. It is often possible to see pulsating arteries in the arms of elderly or emaciated patients.

Note.
It is rare to puncture an artery. However, if an artery is punctured, bright red blood may appear in the sample tube and a haematoma will rapidly appear around the puncture site.

In this case:

- Cease the procedure immediately.
- Put very firm pressure over the site for at least 10 minutes.
- Inform a senior colleague or the medical staff.

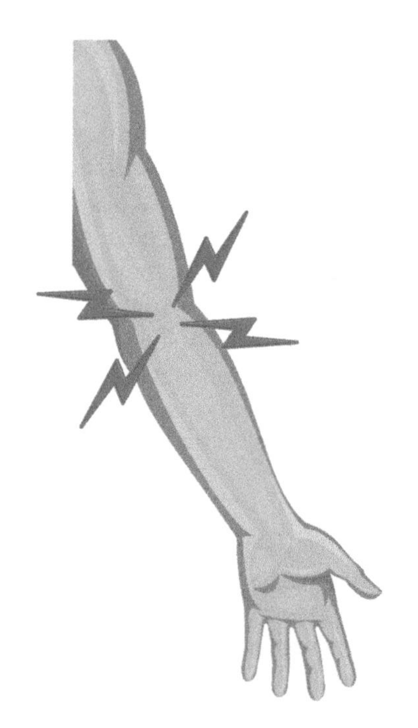

Figure 9. Puncturing a nerve may cause sharp 'lightning' pain, tingling or numbness.

Tendons

Tendons can be deceptive and may appear as veins but they do not feel soft and bouncy and are hard to the touch. Puncturing a tendon gives no blood return and is painful to the patient. To check if a structure is in fact a tendon and not a vein; keep feeling the 'vein' whilst lifting the arm slightly to bend it. Tendons become much more prominent and hard when the arm is bent.

Read your Trust or other Institution's – Adverse Incident Policy

Document Title:

Date: *Signature:*

The Tourniquet

The tourniquet restricts the blood flow in the arm and makes the veins more prominent. The most commonly used tourniquets are the elastic type with plastic fasteners. They usually have a mechanism, which allows the tourniquet to be either slackened or released quickly, whichever is the most suitable.

Sometimes it is in order to slacken the tourniquet without removing it completely so it can be tightened up again if required. Place the tourniquet 3-4 inches (10 cm) above the proposed venepuncture site. It is sometimes helpful to place your fingers under the tourniquet as you tighten it so that it doesn't nip the skin, especially on elderly patients who may have very loose, thin skin.

Pull the tourniquet tight enough to restrict blood flow through the veins but not so tight that it restricts blood flow to the arteries. The radial pulse (in the wrist) should be present throughout the procedure.

The tourniquet should only be tightened for 1 minute to avoid *haemoconcentration* - where the quality of the sample may be affected due to increased concentration of components and chemicals in the blood due to water and smaller components leaking through the vein wall. If left on for longer it also becomes extremely uncomfortable for the patient.

Disposable tourniquets

Many hospitals are now using single-use disposable tourniquets to reduce transmission of infections to patients both through bacteria and blood borne viruses. There is a convincing argument for this but the additional cost will increase budgets. Where these are used either routinely, or simply in isolation units, it is worth taking the time to learn to tie them correctly.

Preparation of the puncture site

Many hospital Trusts have a policy to swab the proposed venepuncture site with a chlorhexidine and isopropyl alcohol swab although this is by no means universal.

Many patients however, expect the skin to be swabbed and find it reassuring. The cost is minimal and every endeavour to prevent healthcare associated infection must constitute 'best practice'.

Prepping the skin is recommended by NAP and the World Health Organisation (WHO).

The 'prep' time is 30 seconds cleaning usually in a spiral motion, and 30 seconds drying time. The cleaning stage mechanically removes bacteria and dry, flaking skin cells and often the swab will look quite dirty afterwards.

This is due to pigment in the skin cells removed during the prep and will be especially noticeable in patients with darker skin.

The swabbed area must be allowed to dry for at least 30 seconds to prevent spirit entering the puncture site. Do not re-palpate the puncture site. If palpation is necessary in difficult circumstances, palpate a little higher than the proposed puncture point.

Phlebotomists often feel the need to re-palpate the vein just before puncturing the vessel. This practise is discouraged as it can re-contaminate the swabbed area.

The procedure for skin cleansing is as follows -

- Clean the area thoroughly with the swab in a circular motion from the centre to the outside. If necessary, use more than one alcohol swab.
- Allow to dry for at least 30 seconds - UNEVAPORATED ALCOHOL STINGS!
- Do not blow or fan the area to accelerate drying time.
- Do not dry with a gauze square.

- Do not ask patients to pump their fist as this concentrates potassium levels in the plasma causing erroneous results.
- Do not slap the arm to encourage veins to appear. Keeping the arm warm helps to encourage the venous blood flow.

Read your Trust or other institution's –
Phlebotomy Policy.

Document Title:

Date: *Signature:*

NOTES

Read your Trust or other institution's –
Adverse Incident Policy.

Document Title:

Date: *Signature:*

NOTES

8. Equipment

The Standard requires you know, understand or are able to do -

18. Working knowledge of the types and functions of the different blood collection systems.

There is a wide variety of phlebotomy equipment in use from three main manufacturers - Becton Dickinson (BD) who produce Vacutainer™ equipment, Greiner Bio-one (Vacuette™) and Sarstedt who produce Monovette™.

Which of these products are used depends largely on the purchasing policy of your hospital or facility.

It is important that you familiarise yourself with each product in your department and understand how to correctly deploy their safety features.

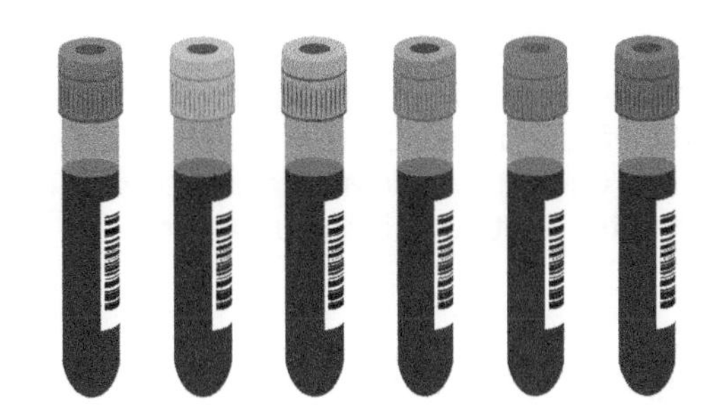

Figure 10. A selection of sample tubes with the coloured stoppers indicating tube additives. These tubes are pre-vacuumed to draw off the correct volume of sample.

Figure 11. Many products already incorporate safety features such as this Vacuette™ holder by Greiner Bio-One. © R.F. Hoke 2015.

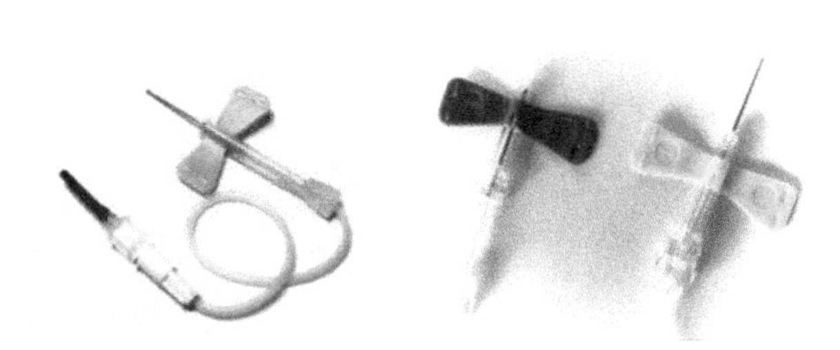

Figure 12. Winged needle blood collection sets from Becton Dickinson (BD) (left) and Greiner Bio-one. © R.F. Hoke 2015

Winged devices are useful for difficult veins as 'flashback' of blood confirms successful venepuncture. They are available in a variety of sizes with safety devices. Whilst many experienced phlebotomists may not require these they are particularly useful for trainees and staff gaining experience and for venepuncture on the back of the hand.

9. Quick Summary

The Standard requires you to know, understand, or are able to do -

19. You have an understanding of what is likely to cause pain or discomfort to the patient.

20. Recognise common events or adverse reactions to blood sampling,and appropriate action to take.

Obtaining a sample

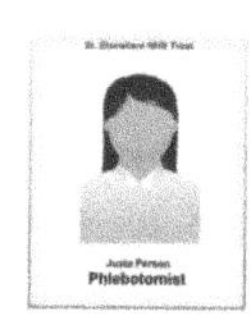

- Introduce yourself to the patient and gain valid consent. Correctly identify the patient by asking them to state their full name and date of birth. Check these details against the identity band (in-patients) or the Request Form if an out-patient.

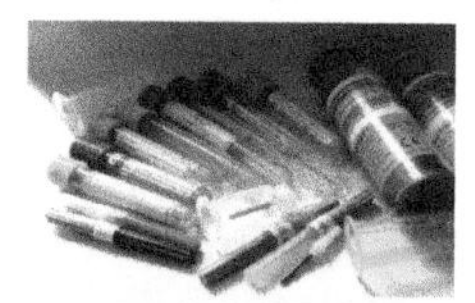

- **Figure 13.** Ensure you have all equipment and sample tubes to complete the request.

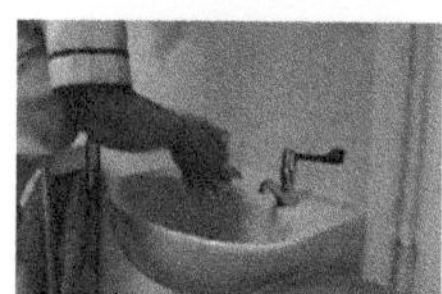

- **Figure 14.** Perform hand hygiene as per your Trust Policy. This may either be hand-washing or applying alcohol gel.

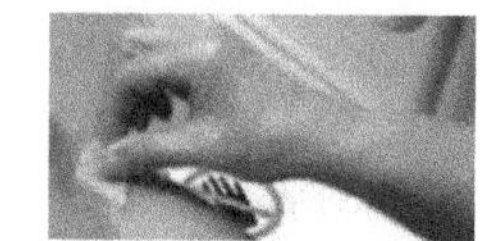

- **Figure 15.** Prep the skin as per your hospital infection control policy and allow site to air dry. This is usually 30 seconds cleaning and 30 seconds minimum drying time.

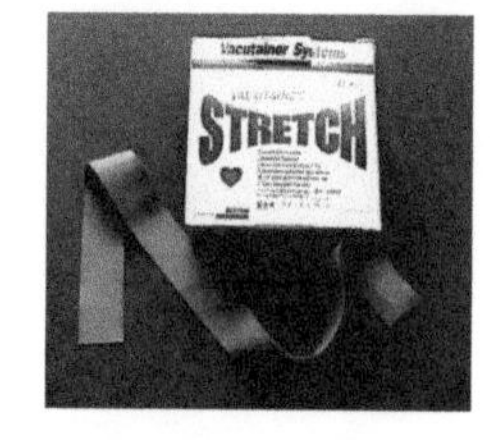

- **Figure 16.** Apply the tourniquet approximately 10 cm above the proposed puncture site. Remember the tourniquet time should not exceed ONE MINUTE. Ensure intravenous infusions are not connected to the arm on the proposed puncture site as erroneous results will occur.

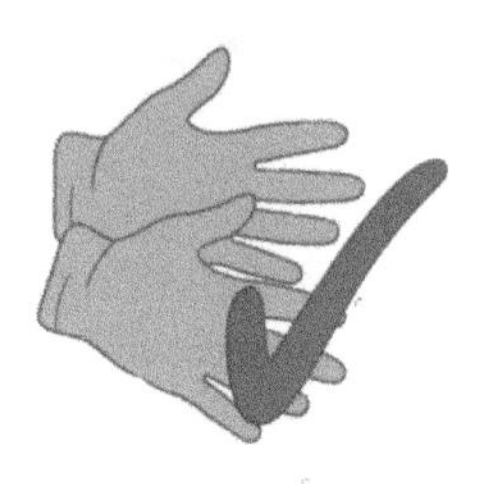

- **Figure 17.** Wear gloves. Avoid latex gloves where possible and remember to consider latex allergies in your patient.

- **Figure 18.** The needle should be inserted at an angel of 15 - 25 degrees depending how near the vein is to the surface.

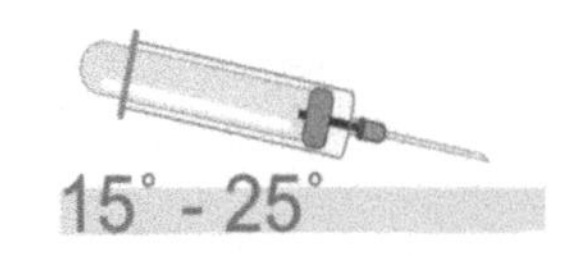

- Always ensure the bevel is uppermost. This reduces pain for the patient and ensures easy venepuncture.

- **Figure 19.** Stretch the skin to stabilise the vein with your non-dominant hand. Insert needle in a straight line directly into vein. Avoid rotating the needle in vein. This allows the needle to cut straight through the skin into the vein quickly, minimising pain and discomfort.

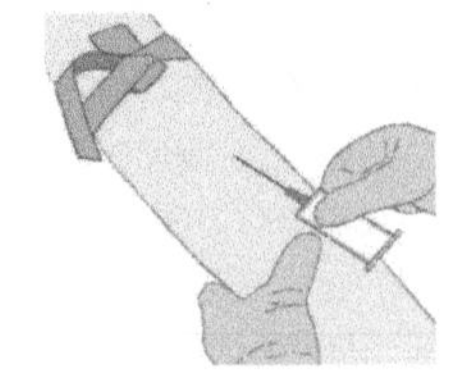

- **Figure 20.** Insert the tube with the label down so that the tube can be observed to fill.

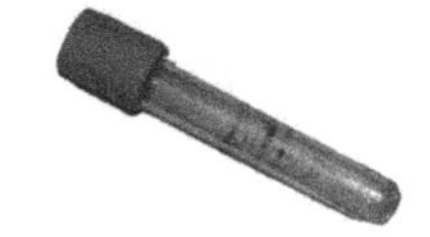

- **Figure 21.** Using the flanges on the holder, squeeze the sample tube onto the multi-sample needle.

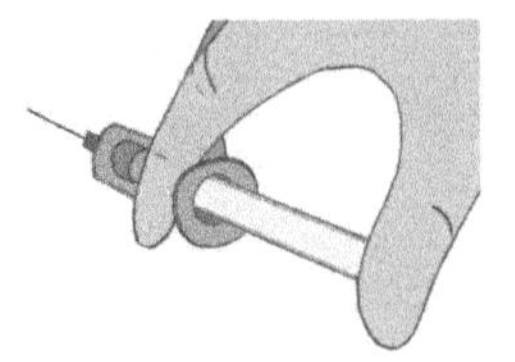

- Release tourniquet when blood begins to flow.

- **Figure 22.** Follow the 'Order of Draw'. Invert tubes 5 - 8 times to mix sample with tube additive.

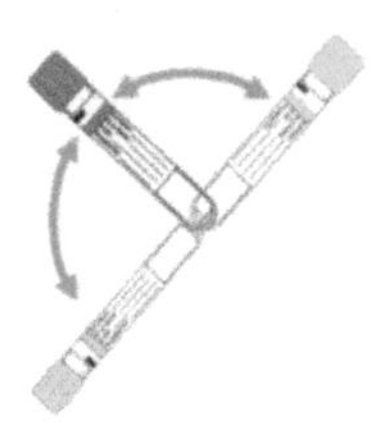

- **Figure 23.** Withdraw needle, activate safety guard and dispose. Apply pressure to the puncture site.

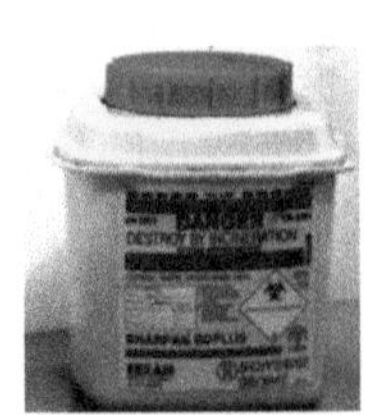

- Apply suitable dressing.

- **Figure 24.** Label sample in presence of the patient and dispatch to laboratory.

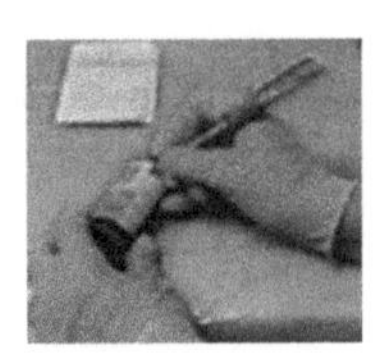

- If further samples are required, take care not to dislodge the needle in the vein.
- Gently pull the tube whilst pushing against the holder.
- Place the swab over the puncture site then remove the needle and apply pressure to the puncture site (or ask your patient to do this) until the bleeding stops.
- Do not put pressure on the site before removing the needle as this causes pain and unnecessary trauma to the vein.
- Throughout the procedure, observe the patient for signs of fainting. Should this occur, lower the head either by placing the head between the knees, or if using a phlebotomy chair, lower the chair to the head down position.
- Dispose of all sharps in 'sharps' container at the point of use.
- Dispose of other clinical waste as appropriate into the correct container following your infection control policy.
- Arrange transportation of the sample as per your departmental policy.
- When bleeding has stopped fix swab in place with Micropore™ or similar tape instructing patient to keep pressure over site for at least 30 minutes.
- Ensure the patient is well enough to leave the clinic.
- Document any adverse effects during the procedure.

The blood sample MUST NOT be taken if: -

- **There is any discrepancy in the identification details.**
- **There is any language or other difficulty such as speech or hearing loss, which prevents proper identification.**
- **The form is incomplete or contains errors.**
- **There is an uncooperative patient.**

Under any of these circumstances, refer the patient to the doctor ordering the test.

Labelling the Samples

It is essential that the samples are labelled immediately with the patient's full name, date of birth, and NHS number or hospital number (if provided).

If samples are left unlabelled they may become confused with samples from another patient.

The samples should be bagged with the appropriate forms and sent directly to the pathology department.

Whilst the patient is applying pressure to the puncture site, the tubes should be labelled as follows: -

- Surname*
- First name in full (not initials) *
- NHS or Hospital number*
- Date of birth (DD-MM-YYYY) *
- Ward/clinic
- Date sample was taken.
- Time sample was taken.
- Signature of phlebotomist (who confirmed patient identification).*

** Mandatory indicators which must not be omitted.*

Never Pre-Label sample tubes

Label blood tubes immediately following the procedure.

- At the bedside / drawing area
- From the Identification Band (where worn)
- By the person who took the sample
- Never use pre-labelled tubes
- Date, time & sign
- Send to laboratory in timely manner
- Keep samples away from heat and cold

Where possible label from the identity band.

Advice to the patient following their blood test;

- Ask the patient not to bend their elbow as this can cause bruising.
- Ask patients not to carry heavy bags or other items for at least 30 minutes.
- Remind the patient to remove the dressing and keep the site clean.
- Advise the patient to report any problems to the ward nursing staff or their GP.

Order of Draw

Blood collection tubes must be drawn in a specific order to avoid cross-contamination of additives between tubes. Tubes with additives must be thoroughly mixed by gently inverting the tube several times.

Erroneous test results may be obtained when the blood is not thoroughly mixed with the additive.

Table 1. The recommended order of draw is:

Blood Culture	AEROBIC
Blood Culture	ANAEROBIC
	Discard tube
	Citrate
	Citrate (ESR)
	Plain tube
	SST
	Lithium Heparin
	EDTA
	EDTA X
	Fluoride Oxalate
	Trace Element

Your Order of Draw where this differs

____

____

____

____

____

____

____

____

____

____

____

____

____

____

The above order may differ slightly to your own department's requirements and may depend on laboratory processes. If you are in any doubt, check requirements with your hospital or laboratory.

Throughout the procedure, observe that the blood flows freely, that there are no signs of a haematoma around the needle entry site, that the patient does not complain of any pain or tingling in the hand or arm, or that they do not feel dizzy or faint. In any of these instances remove the needle from the arm immediately and treat the patient accordingly.

Trouble Shooting

Problem	Cause	Prevention	Suggested Action
Anxiety	Previous trauma or fear of needles	Minimise risk of traumatic venepuncture	Use all methods available to ensure successful venepuncture.
Communication barriers		Ensure patient understands the procedure and is fully informed.	Address communication difficulties before attempting procedure.
Dehydration			May be necessary to re-hydrate the patient prior to venepuncture.
Difficult venous access			Ask an experienced colleague to perform procedure. Observe colleague to gain insight into their technique.
Hardened veins	Due to scarring and thrombosis		Avoid these veins as venepuncture is rarely successful.
Missed veins	Inadequate anchoring or poor vein selection	Ensure only trained staff perform venepuncture or those in training are supervised	Withdraw needle slightly and realign it. Learners should be supervised. Cease attempt if patient is experiencing pain.
Pain	Puncturing an artery	Knowledge of location of arteries	Palpate vessel for pulse. Remove device immediately and apply pressure until bleeding stops. Explain to patient what has happened. Inform patient to contact doctor if pain continues or there is increasing swelling or bruising.

Trouble Shooting

Pain	Touching a nerve	Knowledge of Location of Nerves. Avoid excessive or blind probing. After needle has been inserted.	Remove the needle and apply pressure. Explain to the patient what has happened and that the pain or numbness may last a few hours. Inform patient to contact doctor if pain continues. Provide information leaflet. Document in notes or complete an incident report. Avoid use of vein in sensitive areas (e.g. wrist). Use local anaesthetic cream.
Vaso-vagal Reaction (Fainting)	Fear of needles Low blood sugar Fasting	Spend time listening to the patient and allay their fears	Patients who are known to faint should always be laid down.
Vein Collapsed	Needle too large Or Vein too small		Choose a smaller gauge needle or larger vein

Notes On Competency Assessment

1. Your Assessor must be experienced and be competent in phlebotomy.

2. Ideally, the assessment will look at all components on one patient episode to ensure that all tasks are performed correctly on the same patient.

3. Your assessor may, at their discretion, want to observe you with several patients before choosing one to assess you against.

4. Your assessor should initial against each numbered item when this component has been assessed as satisfactory.

5. On completion, the Assessor should sign the Assessment form confirming they consider you to be competent.

Practical / Performance Criteria

You must be able to do the following -

No.	Date	Description	Assessor Verification
1		Apply Standard Precautions to prevent infection and other health & safety measures including prevention of 'Sharps' injuries.	
2		Provide the patient with relevant information and give support and reassurance.	
3		Identify the patient using Positive Patient Identification methods following national and local policies.	
4		Gain Valid Consent (verbally and implied).	
5		Select and prepare an appropriate venepuncture site.	
6		Select appropriate equipment and sample tubes.	
7		Apply and release tourniquet appropriately, maintaining one minute duration at all times.	
8		Gain successful venous access causing the minimum of pain and discomfort to the patient.	
9		Demonstrate correct selection of sample tubes	
10		Demonstrate correct volume drawn	
11		Demonstrate correct order of draw according to laboratory protocol.	
12		Demonstrate ability to stimulate flow of blood or select an alternative site	
13		Demonstrate prompt identification of any adverse event during or after sample collection.	

No.	Date	Description	Assessor Verification
14		Demonstrate correct use of safety devices on needles and winged collection sets as appropriate.	
15		Provide and maintain haemostasis after blood collection.	
16		Apply a suitable dressing to the puncture site.	
17		Label samples clearly and accurately ensuring all points of ID have been used.	
18		Place sample in correct packaging with correct Request Form.	
19		Place sample in designated place for collection at appropriate temperature and away from direct sunlight.	
20		Ensure urgent samples are transported to the laboratory by appropriate means.	
21		Dispose of all clinical waste as appropriate following national and local policies and guidelines.	
22		Provide advice to patient as appropriate following blood collection.	
23		Complete all documentation as appropriate.	
24		Episode of care completed with hand hygiene.	

Assessors Confirmation of Competence:

Name: ______________________________

Job role or title: ______________________________

Date: ______________ **Signed:** ______________

Courses and Other Training

Date Attended	Course Title	Completion Date	Review Date

Courses and Other Training

Date Attended	Course Title	Completion Date	Review Date

Courses and Other Training

Date Attended	Course Title	Completion Date	Review Date

Glossary

Albumin - a large protein in the blood which acts as a carrier for other substances.

Arteritis - inflammatory condition of arteries.

Arteriole - a small artery connecting arteries to the capillary bed in tissues.

Bacteraemia - the presence of bacteria in the blood stream. *See also septicaemia.*

Capillary - a minute blood vessel in the tissues. The wall of a capillary is just one cell thick.

Cold agglutinin - antibodies which often follow a number of infections and attach themselves to red cells at low temperatures causing haemolysis. Samples need to be kept warm prior to laboratory analysis.

Congenital - a defect existing at birth but not hereditary.

COSHH - *Control Of Substances Hazardous to Heath*. COSHH is the law which relates to controlling and handling hazardous substances.

D-dimer - A fragment resulting from the breakdown of clotting. This is used as a test to indicate clotting such as in cases of deep vein thrombosis (DVT) or pulmonary embolism.

E.S.R. - *Erythrocyte Sedimentation Rate*. A laboratory test based on the rate which erythrocytes (red blood cells) fall and settle in a test tube. The test is used for some infectious disorders especially *temporal arteritis* or *rheumatoid arthritis*.

Embolism - a blockage - usually a blood clot - which has travelled in the circulation and lodged in a blood vessel often in the lung (pulmonary embolism or PE) the brain or veins of the leg. (Plural - emboli)

Haem - the oxygen carrying pigment which gives red blood cells their colour.

Haematoma - Haem (red blood cells) + toma (swelling) a swelling or lump under the skin due to blood leaking from a vein. This
may take several days to a few weeks dissipate depending on the size.

Haemolysis - Haem (Red blood cell) + lysis (breakdown). The breakdown of red blood cells. This releases the red cell pigment haem and potassium into the plasma. Thus, haemolysed samples are not suitable for testing.

I.N.R. - International Normalised Ratio. The standard test for anti-coagulant therapy of the Warfarin type. Internationally standardising the test allows patient on Warfarin to have their blood tested and appropriate medication whilst travelling abroad.

Kleihauer - A test which distinguishes foetal Rhesus D positive blood cells from the mother's Rhesus D negative cells in suspected trans-placental haemorrhage. The test has considerably helped reduce Haemolytic Disease of the New-born (HDN) or 'blue baby syndrome'.

Leucocytes - also known as white blood cells. The role of these cells in to fight infection.

M.H.R.A. - The Medicines and Healthcare Regulatory Authority. This body is responsible for a number of different quality issues surrounding blood transfusion, medicines and equipment. Where there are quality or safety concerns over products, the MHRA issue notifications to healthcare organisations.

M.I. - Myocardial infarction - The medical term for a 'heart attack' or 'coronary'.

N.P.S.A. - National Patient Safety Agency. The NPSA was created by a statutory Act of Parliament to protect patients undergoing healthcare interventions in the UK. It is now part of the NHS Learning and Reporting Service.

P.S.A. - *Prostate Specific Antigen* is used as a marker of prostatic carcinoma.

Platelets - blood cells which are involved in the clotting process.

Septicaemia - the presence of bacteria in the blood stream in sufficient quantities to render the patient 'septic' with fever, headache, malaise.

Thrombocyte - blood cells which are involved in clotting. Also known as platelets.

Thrombosis - the presence of a blood clot(s) within the circulatory System.

Thrombus - a blood clot formed within a vein.

U & E - routine biochemistry tests for urea and electrolytes such as sodium and potassium.

Venule - a small vein which connects capillaries to small veins.

Recommended & Further Reading

1. Hoke R.F. *Phlebotomy*. 2015. Firle & Rose, Portsmouth. ISBN: 978–0-9933140-0-1

2. World Health Organisation. WHO Guidelines on drawing blood: best practices in phlebotomy. http://www.who.int/injection_safety/1card_labTesting_web.pdf?ua=1

3. Skills for Health https://tools.skillsforhealth.org.uk/competence_search/?search=CHS132.

National Association of Phlebotomists
Coldbath Square
London
EC1R 5HL

INDEX

Lightning Source UK Ltd.
Milton Keynes UK
UKHW050855310120
357940UK00004B/35